The Beauty of Food

25 Recipes for Younger Skin without Surgery

Disclaimer and Terms of Use:

Effort has been made to ensure that the information in this book is accurate and complete, however, the author and the publisher do not warrant the accuracy of the information, text and graphics contained within the book due to the rapidly changing nature of science, research, known and unknown facts and internet. The Author and the publisher do not hold any responsibility for errors, omissions or contrary interpretation of the subject matter herein. This book is presented solely for motivational and informational purposes only.

Table of Contents

Introduction

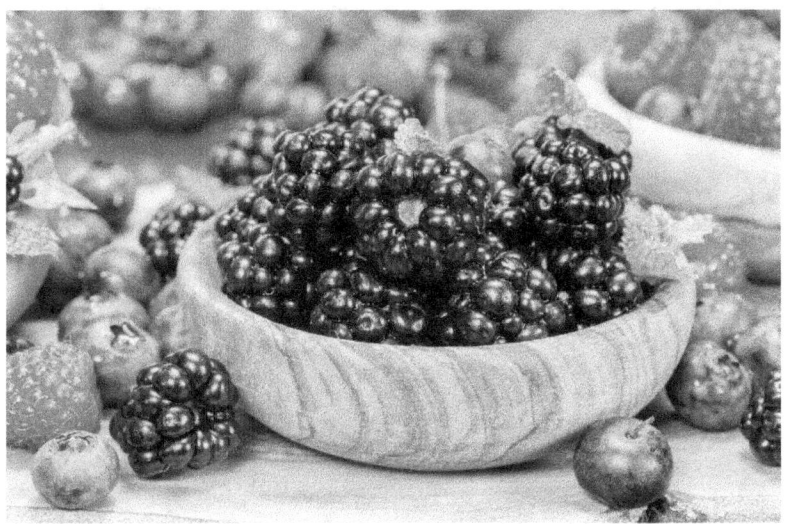

Many people will pay a small fortune just to look a couple years younger, even if it means subjecting their body to invasive surgeries. If you are looking for a way to look a little younger, you will be glad to know that you can do it without surgery – all you have to do is make some simple changes to your diet. You can effectively knock years off of your appearance by making smarter food choices. The foundation of an anti-aging diet is fresh fruits and vegetables, lean protein and whole grains. Adding some exercise to your routine and enjoying a glass of red wine now and then can also boost the anti-aging benefits of your diet. If you are ready to look younger without paying for an expensive surgery, this book is the perfect place to start. Simply pick one of the delicious recipes included in this book and give it a try!

Recipes for Younger Skin

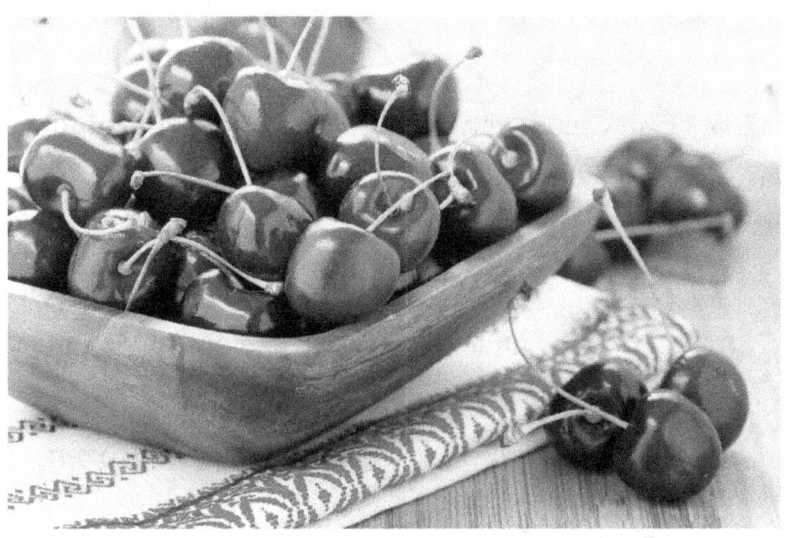

Recipes Included in this Book:

Blueberry Mint Smoothie

Coconut Overnight Oats with Raspberry

Eggs Baked in Avocado

Sweet Green Grape Smoothie

Fresh Fruit Salad with Mint

Spinach Red Pepper Frittata

Tropical Mango Pineapple Smoothie

Curried Carrot Sweet Potato Soup

Apple, Grape and Pecan Chicken Salad

Cinnamon Pumpkin Soup

Easy Egg Salad with Chives

Roasted Acorn Squash Soup

Strawberry Balsamic Spinach Salad

Spring Greens with Avocado and Mango

Balsamic Grilled Salmon

Easy Skillet Steaks

Homemade Meatloaf

Grilled Salmon with Mango Sauce

Vanilla Bean Frozen Yogurt

Peanut Butter Banana Smoothie

Chocolate Chia Seed Pudding

Blackberry Yogurt Protein Smoothie

Chocolate Frozen Yogurt

Creamy Avocado Chocolate Mousse

Chocolate Chia Protein Smoothie

Blueberry Mint Smoothie

Servings: 1

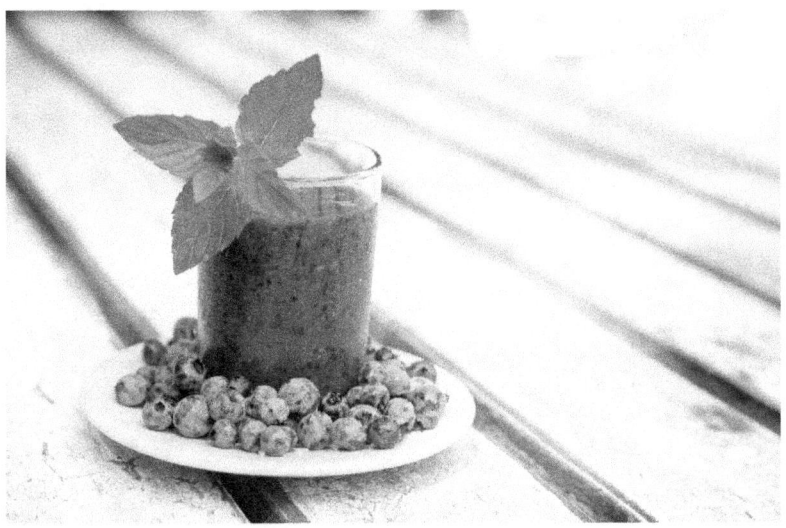

Ingredients:

1 ½ cups frozen blueberries

1 cup skim milk

½ cup plain Greek yogurt

5 to 6 ice cubes

2 tablespoons fresh chopped mint

Instructions:

1. Combine the ingredients in a high-speed blender.
2. Blend on high speed for 30 to 60 seconds until smooth and well combined.
3. Pour into a glass and enjoy immediately.

Eggs Baked in Avocado

Servings: 6

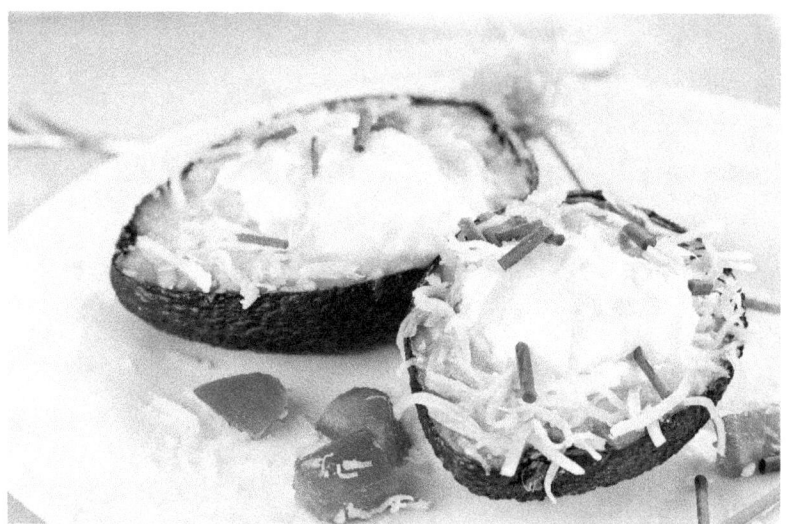

Ingredients:

3 medium ripe avocado

6 large eggs

½ cup shredded cheddar cheese

¼ cup fresh chopped chives

Salt and pepper to taste

Instructions:

1. Preheat your oven to 425°F (220°C).
2. Cut the avocado in half and place them in a glass baking dish.

3. Scoop about 2 tablespoons of avocado flesh from the middle of each half.
4. Crack an egg into each half and sprinkle with cheese and chives.
5. Season with salt and pepper to taste then bake for 15 to 20 minutes until the egg is cooked to the desired level.

Fresh Fruit Salad with Mint

Servings: 6 to 8

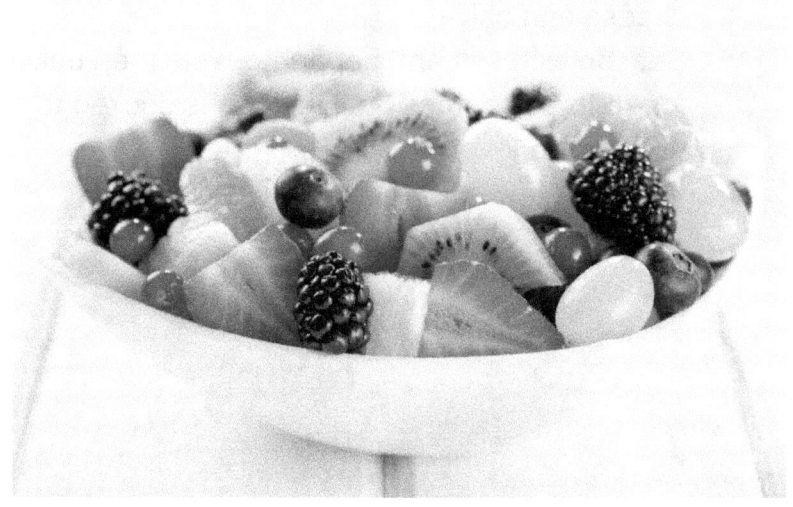

Ingredients:

2 cups fresh sliced strawberries

2 ripe oranges, peeled and chopped

1 cup green seedless grapes

1 cup fresh blackberries

½ cup fresh blueberries

2 ripe kiwifruit, peeled and sliced

¼ cup fresh chopped mint

2 fresh limes, halved

Instructions:

1. Combine the fruit in a large bowl and toss with the mint.
2. Squeeze the limes over the fruit and toss well.
3. Chill the salad until ready to serve.

Tropical Mango Pineapple Smoothie

Servings: 1

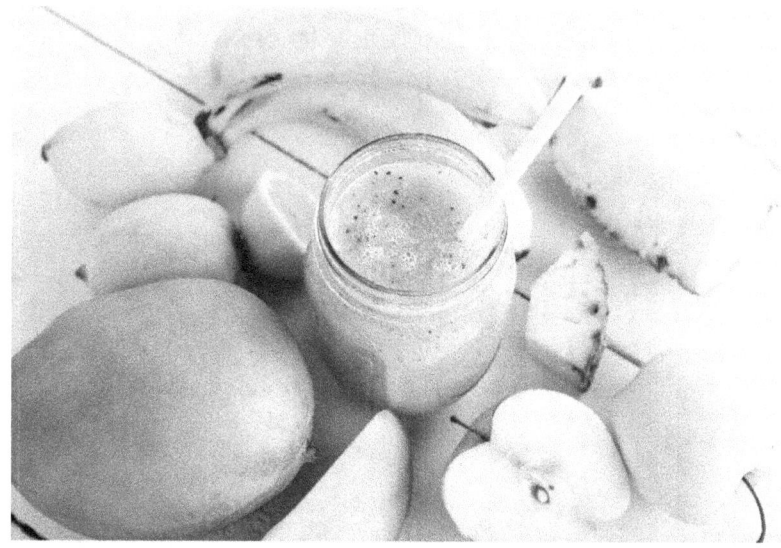

Ingredients:

1 small frozen banana, peeled and sliced

1 cup frozen pineapple chunks

½ cup frozen mango chunks

1 cup skim milk

½ cup plain Greek yogurt

Instructions:

1. Combine the ingredients in a high-speed blender.
2. Blend on high speed for 30 to 60 seconds until smooth and well combined.

3. Pour into a glass and enjoy immediately.

Coconut Overnight Oats with Raspberry

Servings: 4

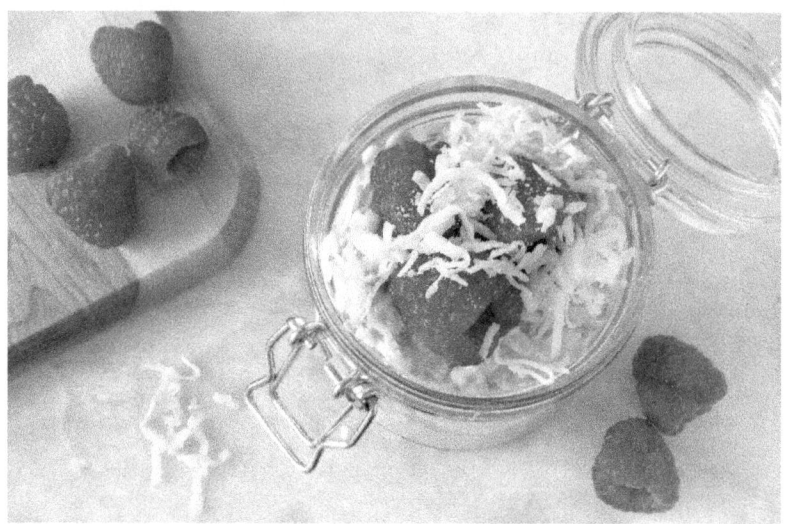

Ingredients:

1 ½ cups old-fashioned oats

1 cup skim milk

2 tablespoons honey or maple syrup

1 ½ teaspoon vanilla extract

1 cup fresh raspberries

½ cup shredded unsweetened coconut

Instructions:

1. Stir together all of the ingredients in a mixing bowl.
2. Cover the bowl and chill overnight.

3. Divide the oatmeal among bowls and top with raspberries and coconut to serve.

Sweet Green Grape Smoothie

Servings: 1

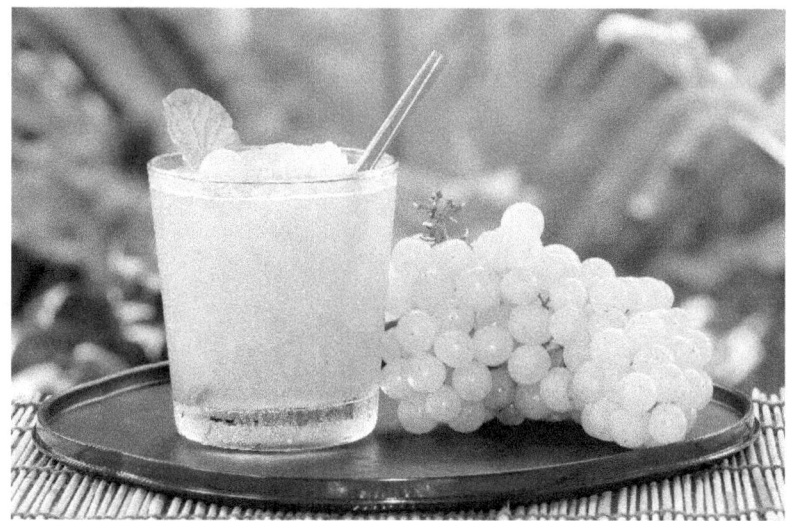

Ingredients:

1 large frozen banana, peeled and sliced

1 cup seedless green grapes

½ cup fresh orange juice

¼ cup plain Greek yogurt

Instructions:

1. Combine the ingredients in a high-speed blender.
2. Blend on high speed for 30 to 60 seconds until smooth and well combined.
3. Pour into a glass and enjoy immediately.

Spinach Red Pepper Frittata

Servings: 6 to 8

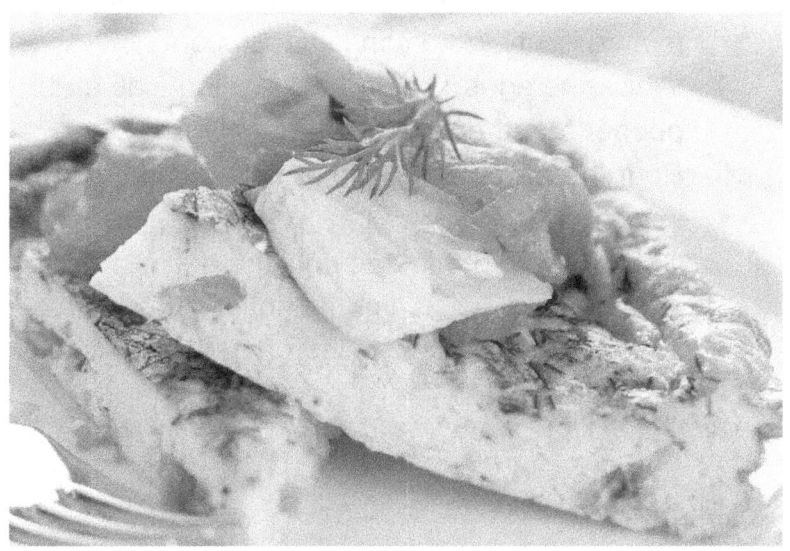

Ingredients:

1 tablespoon unsalted butter

1 large yellow onion, diced

1 large red pepper, cored and diced

10 large eggs, whisked

¼ cup water

2 green onions, sliced thin

Salt and pepper to taste

Instructions:

1. Preheat your broiler to high heat.

2. Melt the butter in a cast-iron skillet over medium heat.
3. Add the onion and red pepper – cook for 5 minutes until the onion is translucent.
4. Whisk the eggs, water, green onion, salt and pepper together in a bowl.
5. Pour the mixture into the skillet –stir in the spinach.
6. Cook for 5 to 6 minutes until the egg is almost set then broil for 2 minutes until the eggs are set.

Curried Carrot Sweet Potato Soup

Servings: 6 to 8

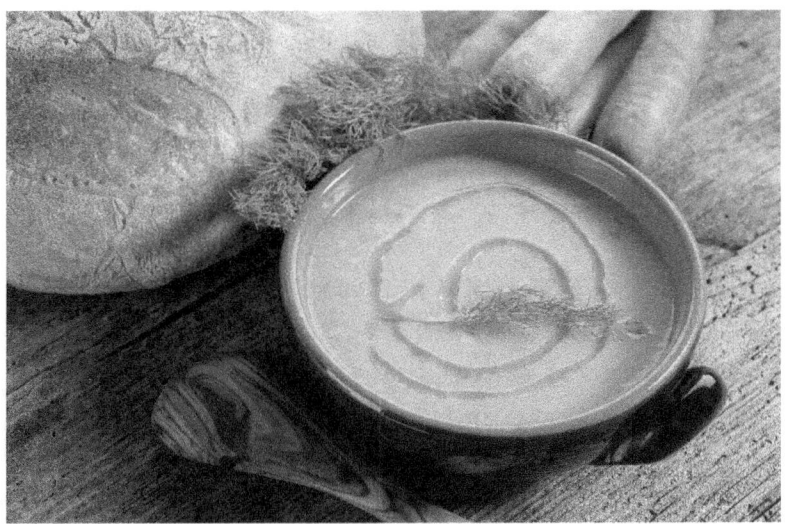

Ingredients:

1 tablespoon olive oil

1 lbs. baby carrots, chopped or sliced

1 large sweet potato, peeled and chopped

1 small yellow onion, chopped

1 tablespoon minced garlic

5 cups chicken or vegetable broth

1 tablespoon lemon juice

1 teaspoon curry powder

Salt and pepper to taste

Instructions:

1. Heat the oil in a large saucepan over medium heat.
2. Add the carrots, sweet potato, onion and garlic.
3. Cook for 5 to 6 minutes until the onion is translucent.
4. Stir in the remaining ingredients then bring to a boil.
5. Reduce heat and simmer for 20 minutes until the vegetables are tender.
6. Remove from heat and puree with an immersion blender until smooth.
7. Season with salt and pepper to taste – serve hot.

Apple, Grape and Pecan Chicken Salad

Servings: 6 to 8

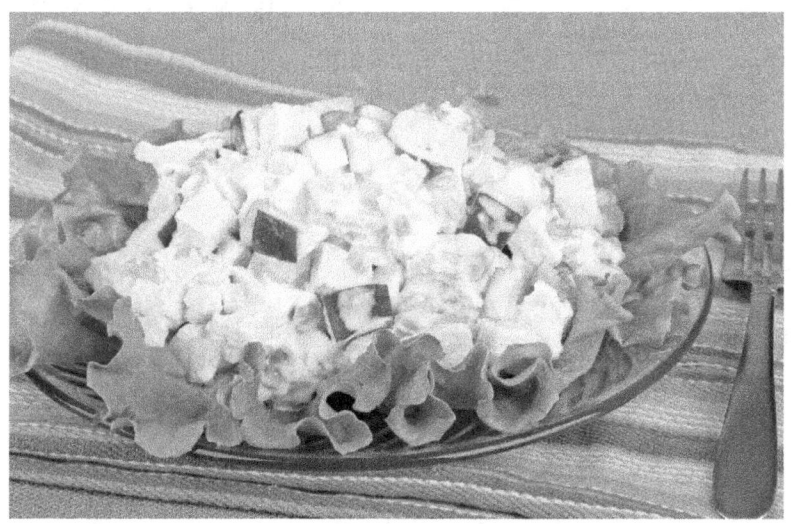

Ingredients:

¾ cup mayonnaise (made with olive oil)

1 tablespoon apple cider vinegar

Salt and pepper to taste

4 cups cooked chicken breast, chopped

2 small apples, cored and chopped

1 cup seedless grapes, halved

½ cup diced celery

¼ cup chopped pecans

Instructions:

1. Whisk together the mayonnaise, apple cider vinegar, salt and pepper in a mixing bowl.
2. Toss in the chicken, apple, grapes, celery and pecans.
3. Season with salt and pepper to taste – chill before serving.

Cinnamon Pumpkin Soup

Servings: 8 to 10

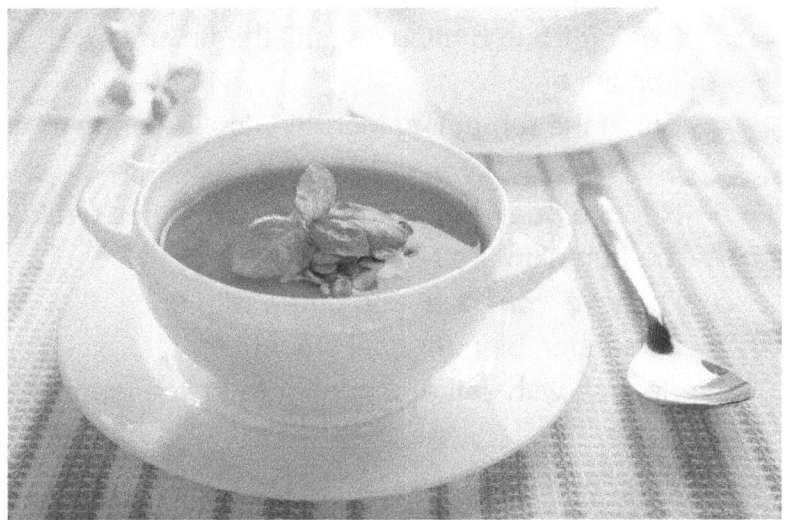

Ingredients:

1 tablespoon olive oil

1 large sweet onion, chopped

2 cloves minced garlic

2 (15-ounce) cans pureed pumpkin

4 cups water

1 ½ cups chicken broth or vegetable broth

1 cup heavy cream

1 teaspoon ground cinnamon

Instructions:

1. Heat the oil in a large saucepan over medium heat.
2. Add the onion and garlic.
3. Cook for 5 to 6 minutes until the onion is translucent.
4. Stir in the remaining ingredients then bring to a boil.
5. Reduce heat and simmer for 20 minutes until the pumpkin are tender.
6. Remove from heat and puree with an immersion blender until smooth.
7. Season with salt and pepper to taste – serve hot.

Easy Egg Salad with Chives

Servings: 6 to 8

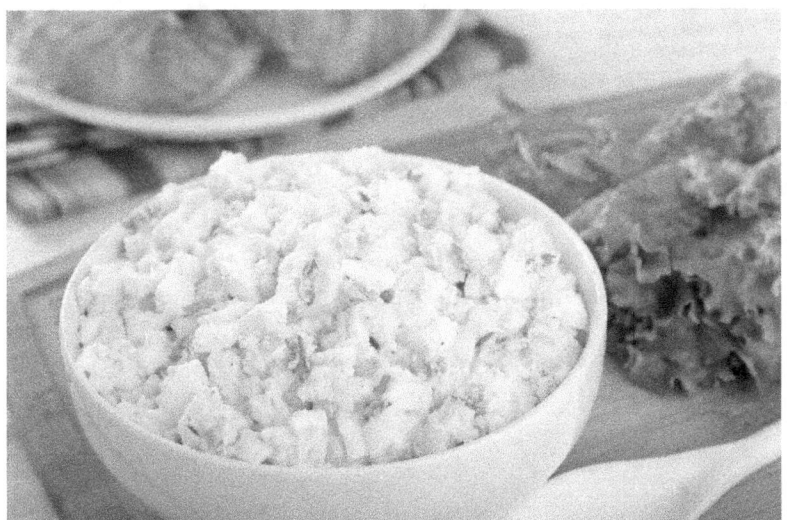

Ingredients:

¾ cup mayonnaise

1 ½ tablespoons Dijon mustard

Salt and pepper to taste

12 large hardboiled eggs, peeled and chopped

2 stalks celery, diced

1/3 cup diced red onion

3 tablespoons chopped chives

Instructions:

1. Whisk together the mayonnaise, mustard, salt and pepper in a mixing bowl.

2. Toss in the eggs, celery, onion and chives.
3. Season with salt and pepper to taste – chill before serving.

Roasted Acorn Squash Soup

Servings: 6 to 8

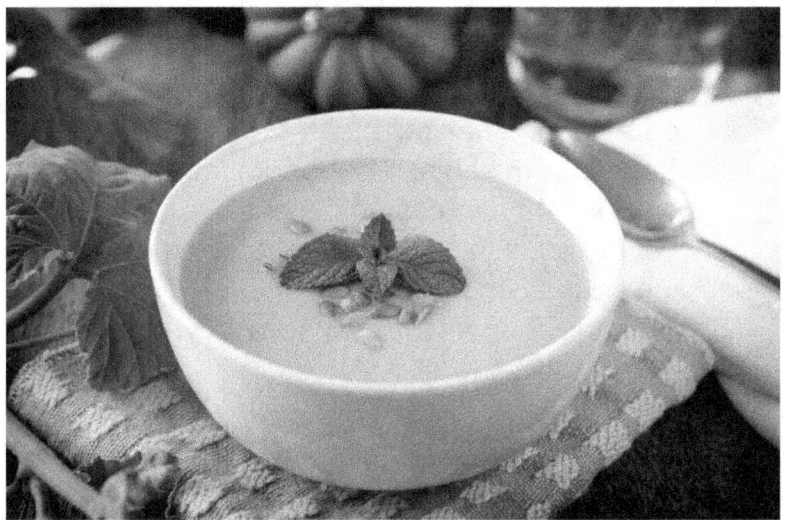

Ingredients:

3 medium acorn squash

2 to 3 tablespoons olive oil

Salt and pepper to taste

2 medium carrots, peeled and chopped

1 stalk celery, diced

1 sweet onion, chopped

1 tablespoon minced garlic

5 cups chicken or vegetable broth

1 teaspoon dried thyme

Instructions:

1. Preheat the oven to 350°F (275°C).
2. Cut the squashes in half and scoop out the seeds.
3. Brush the squash with olive oil then place them on a rimmed baking sheet.
4. Season with salt and pepper to taste then roast for 30 to 45 minutes until tender.
5. Let the squash cool then spoon the flesh out of the squash into a bowl.
6. Heat the oil in a large saucepan over medium heat.
7. Add the carrot, celery, onion and garlic.
8. Cook for 5 to 6 minutes until the onion is translucent.
9. Stir in the remaining ingredients then bring to a boil.
10. Reduce heat and simmer for 20 minutes until the vegetables are tender.
11. Remove from heat and puree with an immersion blender until smooth.
12. Season with salt and pepper to taste – serve hot.

Strawberry Balsamic Spinach Salad

Servings: 6

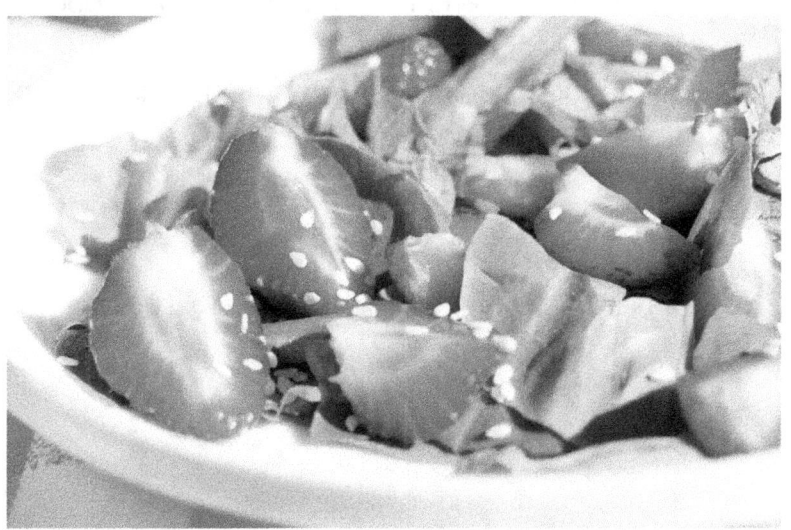

Ingredients:

8 cups fresh baby spinach

1 ½ cups sliced mushrooms

½ small red onion, sliced thin

1 ¾ cups diced strawberries, divided

3 tablespoons olive oil

3 tablespoons balsamic vinegar

Pinch salt and pepper

Instructions:

1. Toss the spinach with the mushrooms, red onion and 1 ½ cups diced strawberries.

2. Divide the salad among six plates and sprinkle with sesame seeds.
3. Combine the remaining ingredients in a food processor.
4. Blend the mixture until smooth and drizzle over the salads to serve.

Spring Greens with Avocado and Mango

Servings: 6

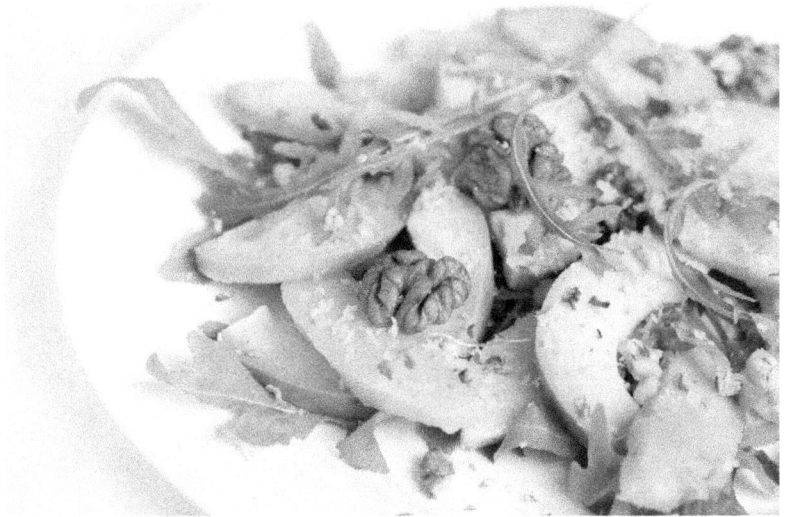

Ingredients:

8 cups fresh spring greens

1 ½ cups sliced mushrooms

½ cup sliced green onion

1 ripe mango, pitted and sliced thin

1 ripe avocado, pitted and sliced thin

¼ cup extra-virgin olive oil

3 tablespoons red wine vinegar

1 tablespoon minced white onion

Pinch dry mustard powder

Instructions:

1. Toss the spring greens with the mushrooms and green onion.
2. Combine the remaining ingredients in a bowl.
3. Whisk the mixture until smooth and toss with the salad to serve.

Balsamic Grilled Salmon

Servings: 6

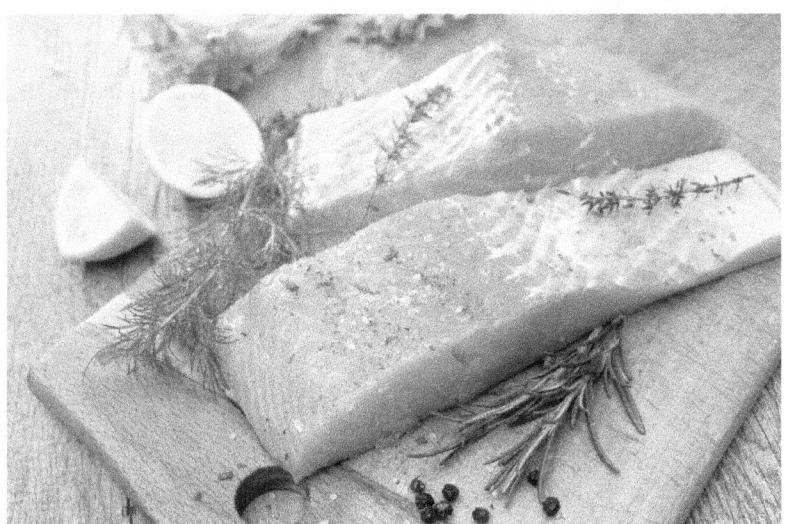

Ingredients:

1/3 cup balsamic vinegar

1/3 cup dry white wine

3 tablespoons fresh lemon juice

2 tablespoons maple syrup

6 (6-ounce) boneless salmon fillets

1 to 2 tablespoon olive oil

Salt and pepper to taste

Instructions:

1. Combine the balsamic vinegar, wine, lemon juice and maple syrup in a saucepan.

2. Bring to simmer and cook for 12 to 15 minutes until thickened.
3. Preheat your grill to high heat and brush the grates with olive oil.
4. Brush the salmon fillets with oil then season with salt and pepper to taste.
5. Place the fillets on the grill and cook for 5 minutes on each side until the flesh flakes easily with a fork.
6. Serve the fillets hot drizzled with balsamic glaze.

Easy Skillet Steaks

Servings: 6

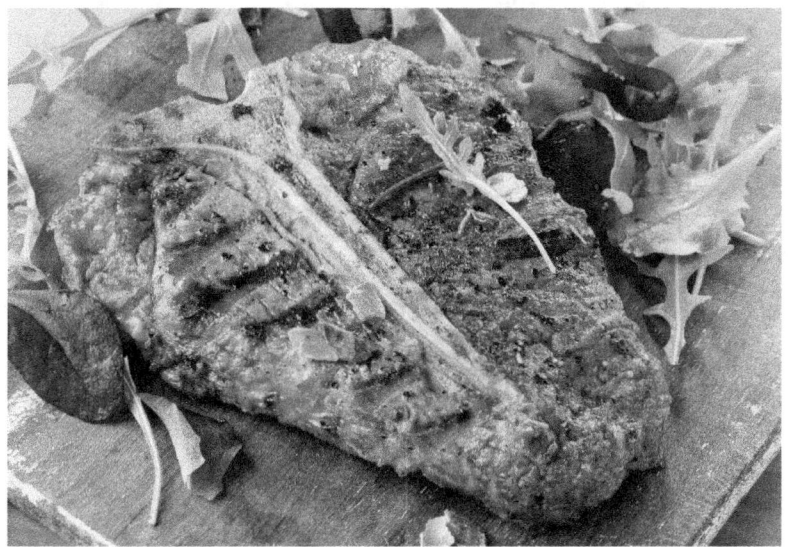

Ingredients:

2 (10 to 12-ounce) New York strip steaks

1 tablespoon coconut oil

Salt and pepper to taste

2 tablespoons unsalted butter

1 tablespoon minced garlic

Instructions:

1. Let the steaks rest at room temperature for 30 minutes before cooking.

2. Heat the oil in a large cast-iron skillet over high heat and season the steaks with salt and pepper to taste.
3. Add the steaks to the skillet and cook for about 3 minutes on each side until browned.
4. Reduce the heat to medium-low then add the butter to the skillet with the garlic.
5. Cook for 1 to 2 minutes, basting the steaks with the butter.
6. Remove from the pan and place on a cutting board.
7. Cover with a tent of foil and let rest 10 minutes before serving.

Homemade Meatloaf

Servings: 6 to 8

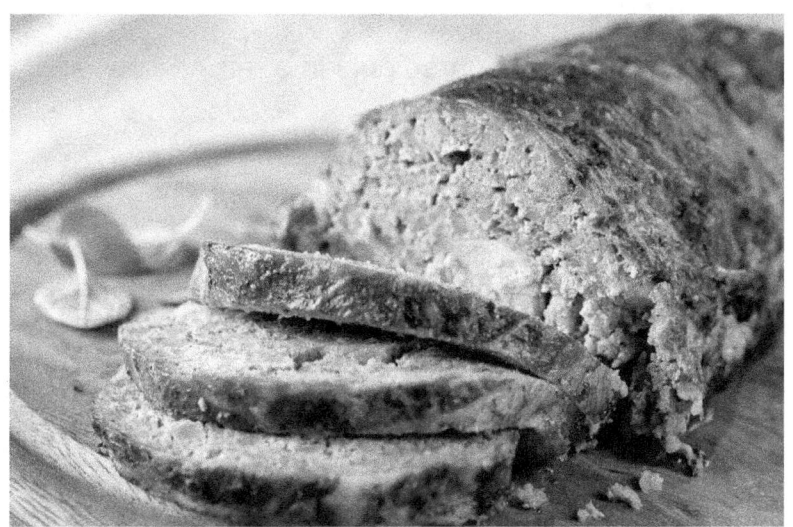

Ingredients:

1 lbs. lean ground beef

½ lbs. lean ground lamb

¼ lbs. lean ground pork

2/3 cup whole-wheat flour

2 large eggs, beaten

¼ cup tomato sauce

2 tablespoons Worcestershire sauce

1 tablespoon Dijon mustard

Salt and pepper to taste

Instructions:

1. Preheat the oven to 400°F (205°C). Grease a loaf pan.
2. Combine the ingredients in a mixing bowl and stir well.
3. Press the mixture into the loaf pan evenly.
4. Bake for 50 to 60 minutes until the internal temperature reaches 165°F (75°C).
5. Turn the meatloaf onto a cutting board and rest for 10 minutes before serving.

Grilled Salmon with Mango Sauce

Servings: 6

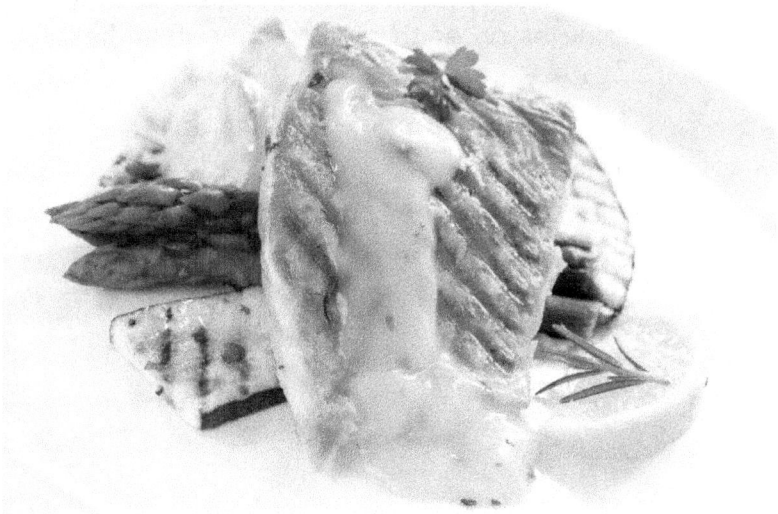

Ingredients:

6 (6-ounce) boneless salmon fillets

1 to 2 tablespoons olive oil

1 ½ ripe mango, pitted and chopped

½ cup canned coconut milk

½ bunch fresh cilantro

Salt and pepper to taste

Instructions:

1. Preheat your grill to high heat and brush the grates with olive oil.

2. Brush the salmon fillets with oil then season with salt and pepper to taste.
3. Place the fillets on the grill and cook for 5 minutes on each side until the flesh flakes easily with a fork.
4. Meanwhile, combine the remaining ingredients in a blender.
5. Blend the mixture until smooth then serve drizzled over the hot salmon fillets.

Vanilla Bean Frozen Yogurt

Servings: 8 to 10

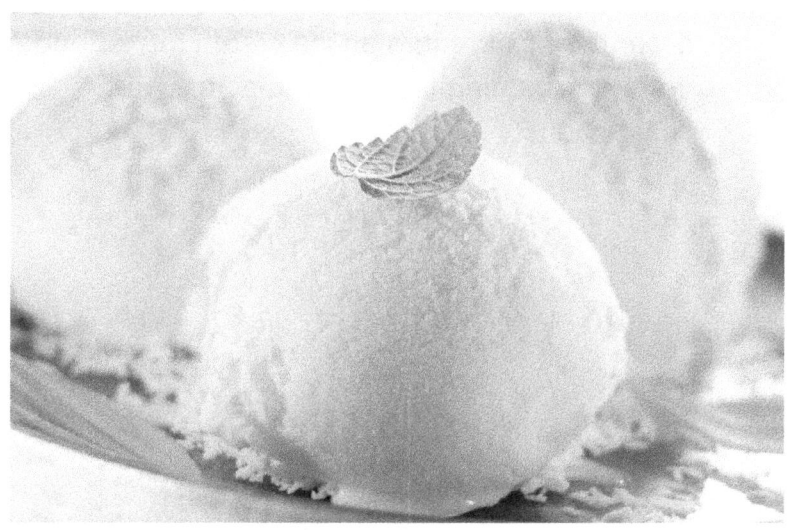

Ingredients:

2 ½ cups vanilla Greek yogurt

2 cups heavy cream

4 large egg yolks, whisked

2 tablespoons vanilla extract

2 fresh vanilla beans, halved

1 teaspoon liquid Stevia

1 tablespoon cornstarch

Instructions:

1. Combine the yogurt and cream in a mixing bowl – beat until soft peaks form.

2. Beat in the egg yolks, vanilla extract and scrape the vanilla bean into the bowl.
3. Whisk in the stevia and cornstarch.
4. Pour the mixture into an ice cream maker and freeze according to the manufacturer's instructions.

Peanut Butter Banana Protein Smoothie

Servings: 1

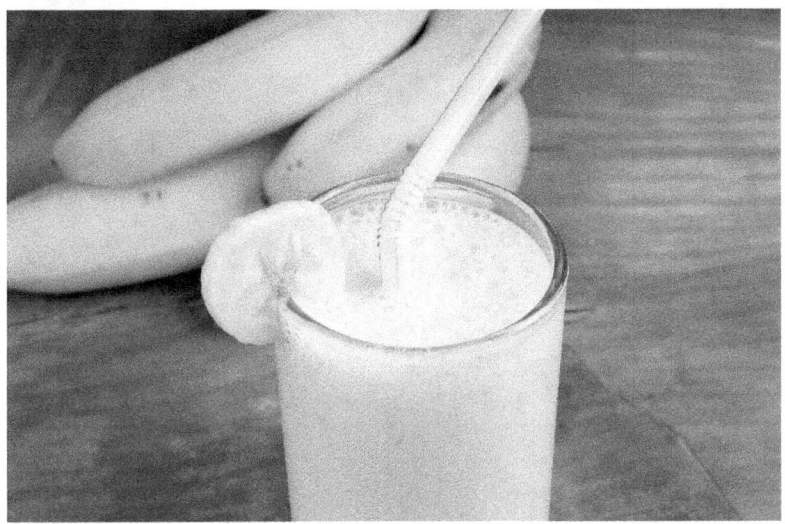

Ingredients:

1 large frozen banana, peeled and sliced

1 cup plain Greek yogurt

½ cup skim milk

2 tablespoons peanut butter

1 scoop vanilla protein powder

Instructions:

1. Combine the ingredients in a high-speed blender.
2. Blend on high speed for 30 to 60 seconds until smooth and well combined.
3. Pour into a glass and enjoy immediately.

Chocolate Chia Seed Pudding

Servings: 6

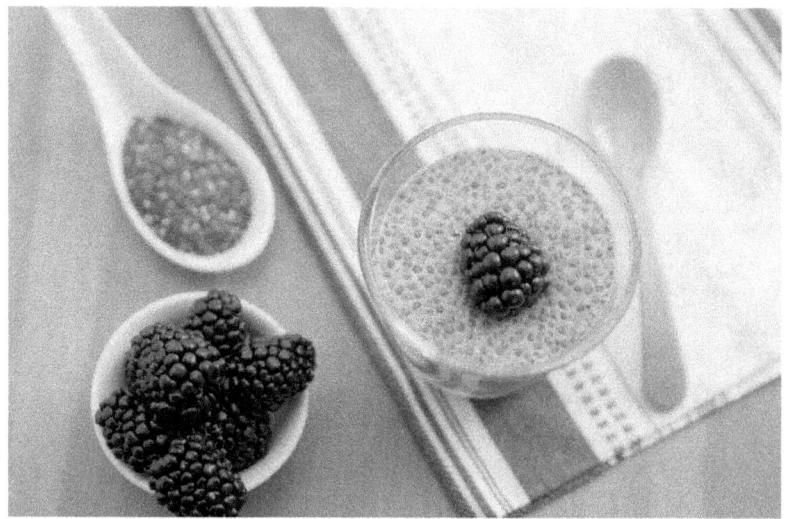

Ingredients:

1 ½ cups heavy cream

1 ¼ cups chia seeds

2 ½ cups skim milk

1/3 cup unsweetened cocoa powder

1 teaspoon liquid Stevia

Instructions:

1. Combine the ingredients in a blender – blend on high speed until smooth.
2. Spoon the pudding into dessert cups.
3. Chill until ready to serve – at least 20 minutes.

Blackberry Yogurt Protein Smoothie

Servings: 1

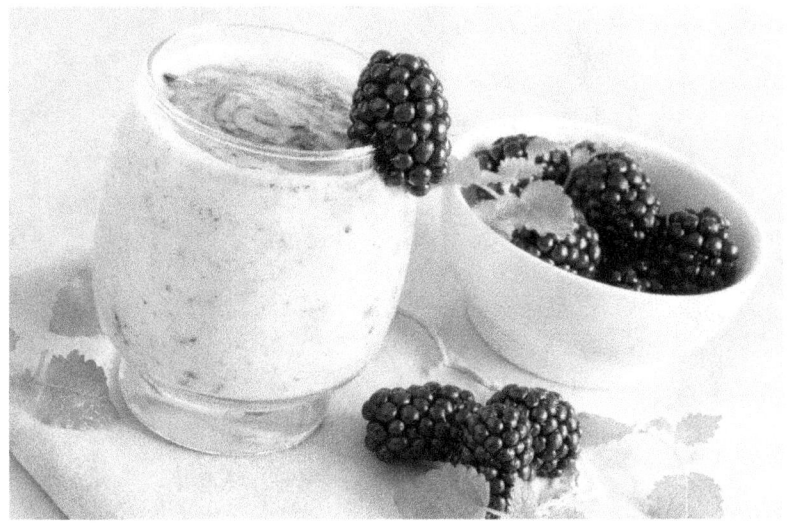

Ingredients:

1 ½ cups frozen blackberries

1 cup plain Greek yogurt

½ cup skim milk

1 scoop vanilla protein powder

1 teaspoon honey

Instructions:

1. Combine the ingredients in a high-speed blender.
2. Blend on high speed for 30 to 60 seconds until smooth and well combined.
3. Pour into a glass and enjoy immediately.

Chocolate Frozen Yogurt

Servings: 8 to 10

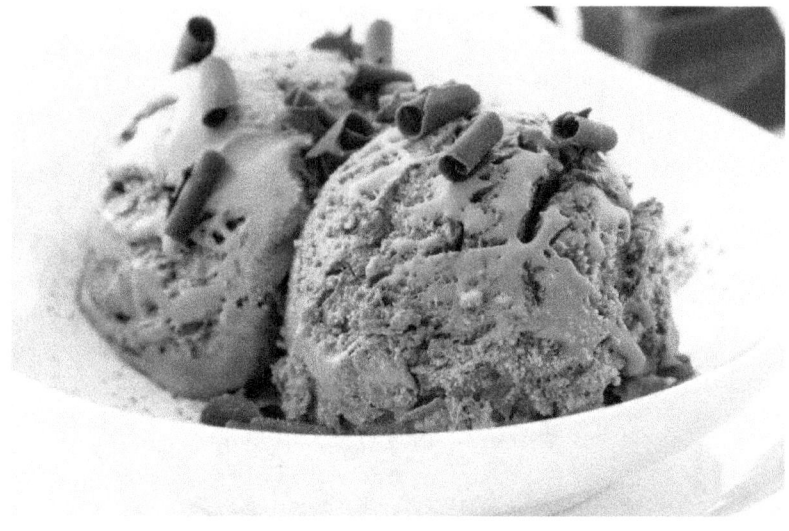

Ingredients:

2 ½ cups plain Greek yogurt

2 cups heavy cream

4 large egg yolks, whisked

1 tablespoon vanilla extract

¼ cup unsweetened cocoa powder

1 to 1 ½ teaspoons liquid Stevia

1 tablespoon cornstarch

1 cup mini chocolate chips

Instructions:

1. Combine the yogurt and cream in a mixing bowl – beat until soft peaks form.
2. Beat in the egg yolks, vanilla extract and cocoa powder.
3. Whisk in the stevia and cornstarch – fold in the chocolate chips.
4. Pour the mixture into an ice cream maker and freeze according to the manufacturer's instructions.

Creamy Avocado Chocolate Mousse

Servings: 4 to 6

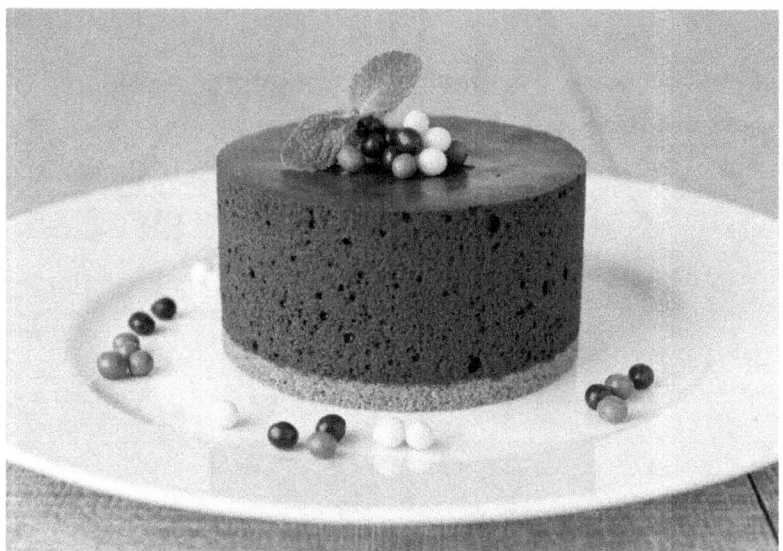

Ingredients:

2 large ripe avocado, pitted and chopped

½ cup heavy cream

¼ cup raw honey

¼ cup unsweetened cocoa powder

1 ½ teaspoon vanilla extract

Instructions:

1. Combine the ingredients in a blender – blend on high speed until smooth.
2. Spoon the mousse into dessert cups.
3. Chill until ready to serve – at least 20 minutes.

Chocolate Chia Protein Smoothie

Servings: 1

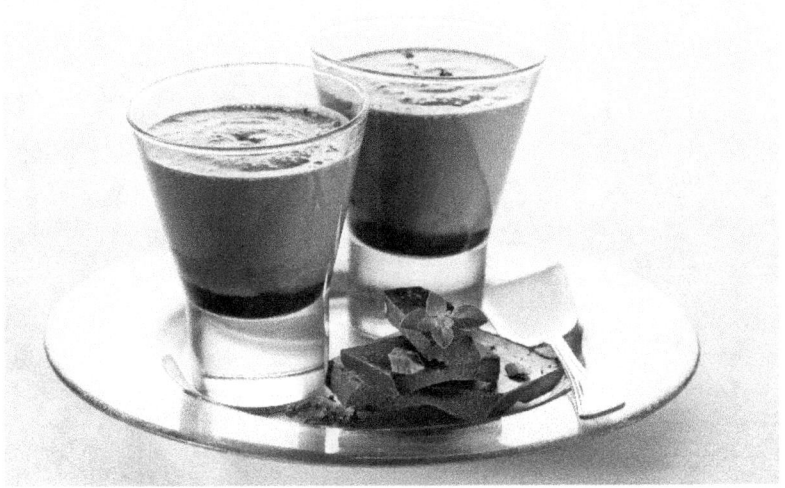

Ingredients:

1 large frozen banana, peeled and sliced

1 cup chocolate soy milk

½ cup plain Greek yogurt

2 tablespoons chia seeds

1 scoop chocolate protein powder

Instructions:

1. Combine the ingredients in a high-speed blender.
2. Blend on high speed for 30 to 60 seconds until smooth and well combined.
3. Pour into a glass and enjoy immediately.

Conclusion

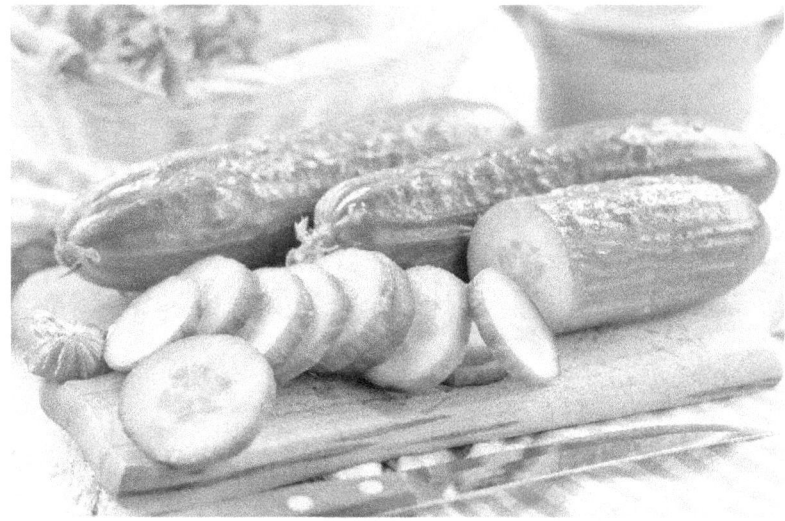

    By making a few simple changes to your diet, you can shave years off of your appearance. The key to looking and feeling younger doesn't lie in expensive plastic surgery, it lies in a healthy diet. The foundation of an anti-aging diet is fresh fruits and vegetables, lean protein, and whole grains. If you are ready to look younger without paying for an expensive surgery, this book is the perfect place to start - just pick one of the delicious recipes included in this book and give it a try!

www.ingramcontent.com/pod-product-compliance
Lightning Source LLC
Chambersburg PA
CBHW070338290526
45791CB00003B/1380